PRINCIPLES OF PSYCHOLOGICAL TREATMENT:

Bruxism & Temporomandibular Disorders

A Research-Based Guide
Fourth Edition

Paula C. Miceli, Ph.D.

The first edition of this book was published in 2014 (ISBN 978-0-9938819-1-6).

This book contains information related to health and health care which is not intended to replace professional medical advice. It is recommended that a health care professional be consulted about your specific health situation. All efforts have been made to ensure the accuracy of information provided in this book. Any use of the information in this book is at the reader's discretion. The author/publisher specifically disclaim any and all liability arising directly or indirectly from the use or application of any information contained in this book.

Internet addresses are provided as a convenience and for informational purposes only. They do not constitute an endorsement or approval of any products, services or opinions of an organization or individual. The publisher bears no responsibility for the accuracy or content of an external site or for any subsequent links. Readers are asked to contact an external site for answers to any questions they may have about website content.

Cover art created with the assistance of stock made available under license from Alliance/Shutterstock.com.
Made in Canada.

ABOUT THE AUTHOR

Born and raised in Hamilton, Ontario, Canada, Paula C. Miceli completed her doctorate in Clinical Psychology at York University. She began her career as a biological scientist, and conducted physiological studies of inflammation-induced neural changes in the gastrointestinal tract. Her interests in clinical research led to a position with a pharmaceutical company, where she led industry-sponsored drug efficacy studies in post-surgical pain and urgency incontinence in Canada. She currently practices as a Clinical and Health Psychologist in the Toronto area. Given the continued integration of psychology in medical settings, one of her goals is to enhance the translation of health-related knowledge for psychologists and mental health clinicians working with medical patients. Her work has been published in journals including *Pain Research and Management, British Journal of Urology International, Journal of Child and Adolescent Psychopharmacology, American Journal of Physiology, Clinical Therapeutics,* and *Autonomic Neuroscience.*

ACKNOWLEDGEMENTS

The author wishes to thank readers for their valuable feedback about this book. Gratitude is also extended to Ms. Lori Santos, B.A. (Hons), B.Ed. and Dr. Jennifer Lewin, C. Psych. for reviewing the first edition of this publication.

PREFACE

It is widely recognized that effective treatment of the pain and dysfunction of Temporomandibular Disorders (TMDs) requires attention to both physical and psychological aspects. One of the difficulties, however, is that knowledge about TMDs rarely reaches community-based psychological practitioners, psychiatrists and other mental health clinicians. Scientific studies are housed in dental journals, or buried deep within textbooks on pain and psychophysiological disorders. At the same time, advances in understanding the stress-health relationship have situated bio-behavioral treatments as first-line therapies for TMDs. Thus, despite the significant role that psychologists and mental health practitioners can play in assisting clients suffering with TMDs, few possess awareness of the condition and its treatment.

The purpose of this research-based guide is to increase the accessibility of health knowledge about TMDs for practicing clinicians. Its format prioritizes information necessary for effective service provision in clinical settings, including symptoms, short- and long-term health outcomes, empirically-supported treatments, and adaptive health behaviors. Such information strengthens the work of community-based mental health practitioners by focusing their efforts towards the most effective intervention targets.

This fourth edition of the book expands its coverage of evidence-based behavioral treatment approaches, with a focus on the efficacy of habit reversal in persons with TMD and/or bruxism. I invite anyone who wishes to discuss their clinical experience in treating TMDs to contact me at TMDprogram@icloud.com.

CONTENTS

TEMPOROMANDIBULAR DISORDERS

Temporomandibular disorders, or TMDs, refer to a collection of disorders characterized by orofacial pain and masticatory dysfunction. Typical symptoms include:

(i.)   pain and tenderness of the masticatory muscles and the temporomandibular (TM) joint (i.e., jaw joint),

(ii.)   popping or clicking sounds in the TM joint during movement of the mandible, and

(iii.)   restrictions in mouth opening and other mandibular movement. [1]

In clinical settings, the primary presenting problem is pain in one or both jaw joints, and difficulties with mouth movements. Pain may also be reported in the neck, back, shoulders, and arms. Earaches, tinnitus, dizziness, and headaches are also common. Mandibular functions, such as chewing, yawning, speaking, swallowing and brushing teeth, are also problematic and/or painful. [2-4]

Clinical examination and differential diagnosis of facial pain and jaw dysfunction is performed by a dentist or physician. TMD prevalence rates vary widely (16-59%) depending upon how it is assessed. Although TMD prevalence is similar in males and females from nonclinical samples, samples of dental clients are mostly female. Signs and symptoms of TMD are believed to be highly prevalent in the general population but not of sufficient intensity to motivate treatment-seeking. [5,6]

TMDs arise due to degenerative or other pathological

conditions of the TM joint, masticatory muscle disorders or a combination of both. Aside from musculoskeletal diseases that affect the TM joint (e.g., osteoarthritis), other contributing factors include tooth malocclusion, physical trauma (e.g., injuries, accidents), hyperactivity/spasm in the masticatory muscles, bruxism, and other para-functional activities (e.g., nail biting, pen chewing). [5,7] The biomechanics of a normal and abnormal TM joint have been illustrated in Glaros & Glass (1993). [5]

Psychosocial Impact

A primary feature of TMDs is the experience of facial and jaw joint pain, and pain-related disruption in daily activities. Dizziness and headaches are also problematic. Persons who experience the problem may refer to their TMD condition using other terms, such as TMJ or TMJ syndrome.

Self-care activities are particularly difficult for persons with TMD. Tooth sensitivity and painful mandibular movements, impact chewing and swallowing food. Social activities involving eating and drinking (e.g., going out for dinner, visiting friends) may also be avoided due to pain, discomfort, and the unpredictability of unusual and embarrassing symptoms (i.e., jaw locking). [2-4]

Occupational and financial strain is also reported. Persons with TMD undergo more frequent and expensive dental therapies (e.g., crowns, extractions, oral surgery), and attend numerous physical therapy appointments to alleviate symptoms. Absenteeism or lack of availability for work is commonly reported. Interpersonal conflict may arise due to the negative impact of teeth grinding noises on a spouse's sleep, a reduction in intimate/sexual activities (e.g., kissing), and financial strain.

The narratives of persons with TMD are compelling. Their stories depict lengthy and stressful periods of searching for a diagnosis, and the need for numerous consultations with different health practitioners to understand their condition. The absence of pathological radiology findings can be distressing for persons with TMD, who fear that they will be dismissed by their physicians and dentists when their symptoms are seen as part of a psychological disorder. [8]

Medical, Dental & Physical Therapies

Surveys indicate that the most common treatments used by persons with TMD include dental, chiropractic and physical therapies. Physical therapies alleviate pain through the relaxation of masticatory muscles, as well as associated muscles of the neck, back, shoulders and head. In addition, physical therapies may alleviate restrictions in mouth opening (i.e., trismus) that occur in association with sustained muscle contraction and/or bruxism. [2]

Medications such as anti-inflammatory agents or analgesics may be prescribed to reduce pain, edema and inflammation in and around the TM joint. Muscle relaxants, anti-anxiety agents and sedatives may be prescribed to alleviate stress. [4,5,9]

Dental interventions include the use of bite guards (i.e., oral appliances) that prevent the teeth of opposing jaws to meet when bruxism occurs. These devices are typically worn while the client is sleeping. Oral appliances reduce the risk of tooth wear, tooth sensitivity, and tooth fracture, but do not alter bruxing behaviors. Dental interventions also address the risks associated with chronic bruxism, including tooth loss, bone loss, recession and inflammation of the gums, and increased risk of periodontal disease. [10,11]

Dental treatments may also include more invasive measures, such as occlusal equilibration, surgery, and orthodontics. Equilibration procedures involve spot grinding of tooth surfaces in an attempt to eliminate discrepancies in the bite. Surgery may be employed in cases of disc abnormality and joint degeneration. [5]

The course of TMDs is usually chronic, and dental, medical

and physical treatments assist with symptom management, but are not curative. Occasionally, persons with TMD enter into a spontaneous remission. [9]

TARGETS OF PSYCHOLOGICAL INTERVENTION

Psychological interventions for TMDs are oriented towards modifying the frequency of oral para-functional activities (e.g., nail biting, pen chewing), reducing hyperactivity and spasm in the masticatory muscles, orofacial pain management, and reducing or eliminating the bruxing behaviors that contribute to masticatory muscle pain.

Oral Para-functional Behaviors:

Para-functional behaviors include biting the lips, tongue, or side of mouth, chewing gum, chewing on pens/pencils, resting the chin and/or side of the face on the hand, thrusting the jaw forward, and holding the telephone receiver between the chin and shoulder. These behaviors are often performed without awareness, which complicates the use of self-report when measuring behavior frequency in clinical and research settings. [12]

TMD treatment recommendations specify that these behaviors should be reduced and/or eliminated. Empirical studies have demonstrated that teeth clenching and resting the hand on the side of the face were positive predictors of jaw joint and muscle pain, accounting for 25% of the variance in pain scores. Caution is warranted about these findings, however, given the lack of validity in self-reported frequency of these behaviors. [7,12]

Hyperactivity & Spasm in Masticatory Muscles

Mind-body theories assert that persons with TMD experience more frequent and intense masticatory muscle hyperactivity compared to non-TMD individuals and that these reactions are a specific muscular response to stress. Masticatory muscles include the masseter, temporal, medial pterygoid and lateral pterygoid, and associated muscles are the sternocleidomastoid (neck) and trapezius (upper back/neck). Empirical evidence has demonstrated that bruxers have a higher resting level of masseter electromyographic (EMG) activity compared to non-bruxers, and a greater masseter EMG activity response to experimentally-induced stress. Bruxers have also been shown to exhibit more frequent occurrences of muscle tension, both in the masticatory system and other regions of the body compared to non-bruxers. [5, 13-15]

Bruxing Behaviors

Bruxism is a nearly universal oral behavior pattern involving gnashing, grinding, clenching, clamping, clicking and tapping of teeth (at times other than when chewing food). The behaviors can emerge at any age, and in persons with and without teeth. Typically, they occur without the awareness of the individual performing it. Instead, the habit is detected by spouses and/or friends who observe the behaviors (clenching) or hear grinding noises at night, and/or by dentists who observe abnormal tooth wear. [9]

In many cases of TMD, bruxing behaviors are related to the onset or exacerbation of tension and pain in the masticatory muscles, as well as the derangement of the TM joint. [16] Mind-body theories assert that persons with TMDs experience more frequent and intense jaw bracing and bruxing behaviors compared to persons without TMD, and that the oral behaviors are triggered by stress. Daytime clenching and/or jaw bracing may occur during stressful situations, and bears resemblance to the guarding and rigidity behaviors observed in patients with chronic pain. Nighttime bruxism is often forceful due to the absence of waking-state cortical inhibition, and lead to tooth damage, gum recession and the need for dental interventions (e.g., crowns, etc.). [3-5, 16]

Accordingly, studies have been conducted to promote awareness and reduction of daytime bruxism. In addition, psychological research has sought to understand the link between bruxism and emotional states. Anxiety, hostility, hyperactivity, emotional stress, panic, reassurance sensitivity, stress sensitivity and abnormalities of mood have been positively linked to bruxing behaviors. [5,13-14,18-23]

Pain and Pain-Related Disability

The alleviation of TMD pain is often a key motivating factor for individuals to seek treatment, and therefore, achieving this outcome is a high priority. Moreover, pain influences the ability to perform self-regulatory and self-care activities, including talking, eating and swallowing, as well as interpersonal and occupational activities. As such, efforts to alleviate pain are vital in the restoration of function. [5]

Some of the interventions for TMD pain are grounded in cognitive-behavioral theories originally developed for use in patients with chronic pain. These theories assert that cognitive and emotional factors influence pain perception and psychological interventions can modify these factors. For example, therapy may include interventions that modify pain reinforcers, reduce emotional distress, and reduce the interference of pain on activities. Strategies for coping with pain can be learned, including attention diversion, imagery training, as well as cognitive re-appraisal of pain-related thoughts and feelings. [5,24,25]

FACTORS RELEVANT TO CLINICAL ASSESSMENT

Psychological Co-Morbidities

Screening for psychological disorders is empirically supported in TMD. Studies have demonstrated that a substantial portion of dental patients with chronic TMD meet criteria for at least one current Axis I disorder (Table 1). Prevalence rates of anxiety and depressive disorders in these samples are substantially higher than the base rates for these disorders in the general population (7% and 2-9%, respectively). [26-30]

Table 1: Prevalence of Anxiety and Depressive Disorders in Studies of Dental Patients with TMD

Study[*]	TMD[**]	N	Depressive Disorder	Anxiety Disorder
Gatchel et al., 1996[a] [26]	Acute	51	12%	47%
	Chronic	50	34%	12%
Kinney et al., 1992[b] [28]	Chronic	50	30%	12%
Kight et al., 1999[c] [27]	Acute + Chronic	277	16%	31%
Korszun et al., 1996[c] [29]	Chronic	51	33%	ns[***]

[*]Various editions of the *Diagnostic and Statistical Manual of Mental Disorders* were used [a=DSM-III; b=DSM-III-R; c= DSM-IV].
[**] TMD is categorized as acute when symptoms are present for <6 months and chronic when symptoms are present for ≥6 months.
[***]ns=not studied

Screening for substance abuse disorders is also warranted in patients with TMD, but the evidence does not suggest a substantially higher risk compared to the general population. In patients with acute and/or chronic TMD, point prevalence rates of substance abuse disorders (2%-8%) were only slightly higher than rates in the general population (3-5%). [26-28,30] Of concern to health care practitioners is that drugs or alcohol may be used to manage orofacial pain. The risk of alcohol use in a sample of orofacial pain patients was shown to be influenced by high pain frequency, being male and being young (i.e., early to mid-adulthood). Marriage was noted to be a protective factor against the use of alcohol to manage pain. [31]

Aside from mental health disorders, clinicians may also need to assess the extent to which psychological factors play a role in the onset, severity, exacerbation and maintenance of TMD pain. The level of psychosocial dysfunction is also important, given that TMD is chronic, and clients may experience disability or other consequences secondary to the pain (e.g., family problems, unemployment). [2,5,32]

Health providers should be alert to the possibility that clients presenting with TMD may not necessarily meet criteria for an ongoing Axis I disorder, but may have experienced a mental health disorder in the past. For example, studies of dental patients with TMD have reported that the lifetime prevalence rates of substance abuse (25-30%), anxiety (24%-53%) and affective disorders (30-45%) are well above the rates in the general population. [26-28]

Dispositional Factors

Personality traits influence an individual's susceptibility to stress-related health conditions. Bruxers have been shown to possess an intropunitive personality style, characterized by fear of expressing anger and frustration externally (to others) and re-directing these emotions toward the self (e.g., internally).

Also, empirical studies with samples of male and female dental patients reveal that bruxers reported greater levels of insecurity, anxiety and tension on the Cattell 16 Personality Factor Questionnaire compared to non-bruxers. [11,33]

Dispositional coping styles are also relevant because they refer to generalized ways of behaving in stressful situations that are stable over time and across circumstances. Compared to non-bruxers, bruxers reported lower levels of adaptive responses to stress (positive coping strategies) on the Stress Coping Questionnaire. The frequency of negative coping strategies (e.g., avoidance, escape) was similar between the two groups. The results suggested that bruxers tended to experience a loss of control with respect to their own stress response, self-encouragement was uncommon, and when they compared themselves to others, they had less confidence in their own resources. In stressful situations, bruxers reported that they rarely used distraction and tended not to use recreational involvement to alleviate tension. [34]

The presence of Axis II disorders influences how persons with TMD manage their illness, and can complicate the course of medical, dental and psychological treatments. In studies of TMD patients, point prevalence rates of Axis II disorders were reported in the range of 29% to 40%, with highest rates in the paranoid (7-18%), obsessive-compulsive (10-22%), histrionic (8%) and borderline (10%) types. These rates are larger than base rates, which fall below 3%. Since longitudinal studies have not been conducted, it is not possible to ascertain whether Axis II disorders develop as a cause or consequence of TMD. [26-28,30]

Screening for Psychotropic Medications

Bruxing behaviors are a known side effect of some psychotropic medications (e.g., SSRIs, antipsychotics, antidepressants). Knowledge about clients' use of these medications is valuable, given that medication-induced bruxism is unlikely to abate with psychological interventions.

EVIDENCE-BASED APPROACHES TO PSYCHOLOGICAL TREATMENT

Bio-behavioral treatment modalities have been shown to be safe and effective in managing the pain and dysfunction of TMDs. These methods promote the restoration and maintenance of psychosocial function and engage the clients' sense of self-efficacy in managing their condition. In this section, information about these modalities is provided, including behavior therapy (habit reversal), EMG biofeedback, cognitive-behavioral therapy, relaxation, psycho-education and hypnosis. Within each modality, emphasis is placed on the rationale of the approach, length of treatment, theoretical basis, and efficacy.

HABIT REVERSAL

Habit reversal is a behavioral treatment approach developed in the 1970s to treat motor/vocal tics, stuttering and nervous habits, such as nail-biting and hair pulling. [35] Azrin & Nunn (1973), who developed the approach, proposed the use of ten interventions that fall into five broad categories: symptom recording, awareness training, competing response training, motivational enhancement, and generalization training. [36] The first application of Azrin and Nunn's approach to treat jaw-related symptoms (e.g., grinding, clenching, popping) in adults with bruxism emerged in the 1980's. [37] Studies on the effect of habit reversal on facial pain in adult TMD patients were published in the decade that followed. [16,38] A summary of the research studies is given in Table 2.

The theory underlying the use of habit reversal is that oral movements (teeth grinding, clenching) are stress reactions that increase in frequency and become automatic (i.e., a habit). In the early stages, one is not aware of stress-related movements of the jaws and teeth, and they blend easily into other movements. As such, they are not perceived as inconvenient or unusual, and are not intentionally held back or suppressed by the person performing them. [36] At the same time, positive effects, such as tension reduction, may be experienced with the movements. In later stages, the activities of the muscles blend into one whole movement or "response chain", which also occurs without awareness. Social reinforcement, in the form of sympathy or attention, may maintain the response chain. [39] Habit reversal treatment was developed to reduce the frequency of these stress-based jaw and teeth movements. The essential therapeutic targets are:

(i.)   awareness of the habit as it happens
(ii.)   interruption of the habit (i.e., break the "response chain")
(iii.)   initiation of a physically competing response to interfere with the habit and strengthen an opposing (antagonistic) group of muscles, and
(iv.)   reversal or elimination of social reinforcement.

It is beyond the scope of this section to fully describe each of the habit reversal interventions. Readers are invited to review Azrin and Nunn (1973) or Rosenbaum and Ayllon (1981) for in-depth descriptions. [36,37]

Summary of the Studies Examining the Efficacy of Habit Reversal in Adults with Temporomandibular Disorder[1]

Study	Design (n)[2]	Components of Habit Reversal Protocol	Primary Study Outcome[2]
Rosenbaum & Ayllon (1981) [37]	Case report (4) HR vs. baseline	-Symptom Recording -Awareness training -Competing response training -Generalization training -Relaxation/Stress Management[3]	Facial Pain (2) Jaw popping (1) Grinding (1) Clenching (2)
Peterson et al. (1993) [16]	Case report (3) HR vs. baseline	-Symptom Recording -Awareness training -Competing response training	Facial pain CDI[4]
Gramling et al. (1996) [38]	RG HR (9) Vs. No-treatment (7)	-Symptom Recording -Awareness training -Competing response training -Progressive muscle relaxation & deep breathing -Identify and reverse maladaptive cognitions -Positive coping statements	Facial pain
Townsend et al. (2001) [41]	RG HR (10) vs. Wait-list control (10)	-Symptom Recording -Awareness training -Competing response training -Progressive muscle relaxation -Deep breathing	Facial pain
Glaros et al. (2007) [40]	RG HR (4) vs. Modified Splint Therapy (4)	-Symptom Recording -Awareness training -Competing response training (including biofeedback)	Facial pain

[1]All studies included adults with TMD except [36] which recruited adults with bruxism; [2]HR=habit reversal; RG=randomized group; (n)= no. of participants; [3]only 2 of 4 participants received this intervention; [4]CDI= Craniomandibular Dysfunction Index.

Both controlled studies and case studies support the use of habit reversal as a effective behavioral treatment for facial pain in adults with TMD. [16,38,40,41] Reductions in facial pain ratings were observed after 4 to 6 weeks of treatment, and maintained at a 3-month [16], 8-month [41] or 1-year [40] follow-up assessments. There was evidence of treatment non-response in one participant in a case study. [16]

Only one study (i.e., a case report) examined the impact of habit reversal on daytime frequency of jaw-related symptoms (e.g., grinding, clenching, popping) in adults. [37] Clinically significant symptom reduction was reported after 1 month of treatment (53% to 99%) compared to baseline. It is worthy to note that one participant experienced appreciable reductions in clenching (-84%) but minimal changes in facial pain (+4%). Addition of relaxation and stress management interventions led to further reductions in both teeth clenching and facial pain ratings.

Treatment protocols were highly variable in terms of content, duration, and level of therapist contact. None of the studies incorporated all five categories of Azrin and Nunn's original protocol. [36] In addition, four of the five studies augmented the habit reversal protocol with other interventions (i.e., biofeedback, cognitive strategies, relaxation/stress management). Treatment usually involved weekly therapist contact, and fell between 4 to 20 sessions in length. Two studies employed a "minimal therapist contact" model, where participants were either given a self-help manual to work through [41] or were paged on a schedule to prompt awareness of muscle tension and encourage use of competing response strategies. [40]

BIOFEEDBACK THERAPY

Biofeedback therapy involves the use of recordings from the masticatory muscles (masseter, temporalis) to modify tension and reduce bruxism. Numerous controlled studies have supported electromyographic (EMG) biofeedback as a highly effective treatment in reducing bruxism. The beneficial effects are generally considered to be limited to TMD patients who have masticatory muscle pain and dysfunction symptoms, rather than joint pathology. [9,50,53,54]

Treatment protocols are typically six to eight sessions in length and conducted on a weekly or bi-weekly schedule. Various treatment protocols are used. One method provides EMG feedback to clients by way of a continuous audible tone that signifies the level of muscular tension, and is performed while in-session with the therapist. Clients are invited to induce relaxation, and can monitor their progress with changes in the tone as the session unfolds. A second approach, the Conditioning Approach, requires patients to be attached to the EMG device before retiring to bed, and when a pre-determined masseter muscle activity threshold is reached, they are awakened by an alarm. The alarm interrupts nocturnal bruxing activities and brings the event to the awareness of the client. Both protocols have been demonstrated to effectively reduce pain and/or the rate and duration of nocturnal bruxism. [3,10,11,55,56]

One of the observed limitations of the Conditioning Approach is that when the arousal stimulus is removed, nocturnal bruxism partially returns. Overcorrection procedures were introduced as a means to achieve better effectiveness with the method. Overcorrection involves the use of a positive practice (e.g., brushing teeth) before returning to sleep in order for the patient to achieve full arousal from sleep after hearing the nocturnal alarm. Case studies offered empirical evidence that arousal with overcorrection successfully eliminates nocturnal bruxism over an 18-month post-treatment period. Moreover, intermittent schedules of arousal with overcorrection have been suggested once the frequency of nocturnal bruxism becomes stabilized. [10,11]

Surprisingly, there are few studies targeting the problem of daytime bruxism, and whether a primary EMG-based intervention in daytime bruxism may generalize to nocturnal bruxism. Moreover, while successful treatment presumes that TMD patients generalize the treatment response to everyday life, there has been little examination of the factors contributing to generalization of the initial positive treatment response. Regrettably, research interest in EMG biofeedback has waned over time, and there are few studies in the recent research literature on this topic. [9,53]

COGNITIVE-BEHAVIORAL THERAPY

Prospective, controlled studies have supported the use of cognitive-behavioral therapy (CBT) to alleviate TMD pain. CBT interventions are a flexible set of tools employed by therapists while working with groups or individuals. In clinical studies, the efficacy or CBT has been tested using groups and standardized protocols. These protocols included pain logs (self-monitoring), cognitive re-appraisal strategies, and coping/stress management skills. Other therapeutic elements were also incorporated into the protocols, such as jaw exercises, relaxation therapy with/without EMG feedback or hypnotic interventions. [24,25,56,57]

There are no present recommendations regarding the number of CBT sessions required to produce a lasting remediation of pain in TMD patients. Efficacy has been demonstrated in studies employing regimens of four or six sessions in length, as well as 15-20 sessions. A brief CBT intervention of 2 sessions have been shown to be a useful adjunct to dental treatment (e.g., oral appliance therapy). All studies reported longer-term therapeutic gains at 3 months and 1 year post-treatment. Reductions in anxiety and somatization were also reported. [24,25,53,56,57]

Studies have also demonstrated that CBT is a cost-effective treatment modality, because patients with chronic pain who received CBT attended significantly fewer medical visits in the year following treatment. [53]

A limitation of the CBT approach is that it focuses on

alleviation of pain, and does not address the frequency or intensity of bruxing behaviors, which contributes to pain and jaw-related dysfunction.

RELAXATION TECHNIQUES

Stress have been recognized as a potent cognitive and affective factor influencing the experience of pain, as well as being involved in the initiation and maintenance of bruxing behaviors and masticatory muscle hyperactivity/spasm. Relaxation techniques refer to a series of activities undertaken by the patient to enter into a full-body state that reduces the tone of the sympathetic nervous system, relieves stress and promotes a sense of well-being. In psychological settings, the technique typically refers to the instructions for standard progressive muscle relaxation, such as those in Jacobson`s original work, or more contemporary works. Relaxation training can also refer to other activities, such as Restorative Yoga or Yoga Nidra, which are based in Eastern philosophies. [24,50-52]

Current models of therapy incorporate relaxation training into a comprehensive bio-behavioral treatment plan, rather than as a stand-alone therapy. Empirical studies have demonstrated that relaxation combined with cognitive behavioral therapy (i.e., cognitive coping strategies for pain) effectively reduce TMD pain after four weekly sessions. [24,53]

PSYCHOEDUCATION

There are several areas in which education can be of value to clients undergoing psychosocial treatment for TMD.

Information about the health risks of combining alcohol with pain medications is empirically supported and likely to be of benefit due to the chronicity of the condition. Health risks of alcohol consumption with pain medications include gastrointestinal bleeding, hepatotoxicity, respiratory depression, and sedation. [22, 24]

In addition, advice about behaviors that may increase jaw joint and muscle pain is also an important aspect of psychoeducation. For example, hard and chewy foods and other para-functional behaviors (e.g., chewing gum, ice, pens, pencils) are to be avoided. Deliberate cracking or popping of the jaw joint is also maladaptive in the long-term. [5,7]

Lastly, information about the musculature of the head, neck, shoulder, jaws and back (including pictures), as well as instructions about stretching exercises, are helpful in pain management.

HYPNOSIS

As a treatment modality, hypnosis involves a variety of interventions. While in-session, a hypnotic induction is used to facilitate a state in which the client is open to therapeutic ideas, and suggestions are made to re-orient the client to the problem. Suggestions may be given to reduce pain and cultivate comfort (relaxation) through association to cues in everyday life. In addition to these sessions, clients may receive instructions about how to perform self-hypnosis, or to use tape recordings to facilitate self-hypnosis in their home environment. [42,43]

Case reports have documented the successful elimination of bruxism habits and jaw joint pain, as well as "hysterical trismus". Trismus, commonly known as "lockjaw", is an inability to open the mouth due to muscular spasm and can be stress-related. [44-48]

Prospective, controlled clinical trials have supported the use of hypnotic interventions to alleviate pain symptoms in the TM joint and to improve psychosocial function. Treatments were offered in a group format at weekly intervals for six or seven weeks, and included daily home practice of self-hypnosis. A recent study demonstrated the effectiveness of hypnotic interventions integrated into a cognitive-behavioral treatment protocol to treat pain in TMD patients vs. conservative treatment (eg., splint use, jaw/neck exercises, use of anti-inflammatory drugs and/or muscle relaxants for pain). Efficacy was evaluated using measures of self-reported pain rather than masseter muscle tension/activity. [4,25,49]

One of the concerns with respect to hypnosis is the ability to generate a sustained effect over time. In this respect, case reports regarding bruxing behaviors have been variable. Five-year remission has been described in a 63-year old woman with a lengthy history of bruxism. On the other hand, relapse of bruxism has been reported following a six-month remission in a 17-year old woman. With respect to pain and daily function, clinical trials have reported maintenance of clinical outcomes for at least 6 months post-treatment. [4,45,46]

Hypnotic interventions are best handled by certified therapists who have undergone training and education in this modality. Concerns about the lack of standardization in hypnotic inductions and interventions have been raised. In clinical settings, therapists rely upon their own judgment, prior training and experience, and professional resources. [43]

Published articles affirm that hypnotic interventions are most beneficial when clients are cooperative and motivated to participate. Contraindications to hypnosis include (but may not be limited to): severe psychopathology, severe interpersonal distress or psychosocial stressors, or evidence of secondary gain. Such exclusions are not permanent, however. Studies have indicated that other forms of psychotherapy may be utilized to address these types of problems prior to the use of hypnotic interventions. [44]

TREATMENT-RELATED ISSUES

Medical & Dental Evaluation

In psychological clinics, clients seeking treatment for

masticatory muscle pain and dysfunction (TMDs) are often referred from medical and dental specialists. However, community-based mental health clinicians may encounter clients who self-refer for mental health concerns and later report masticatory and/or TM joint pain and dysfunction symptoms. Such clients should be encouraged to undergo an evaluation by a dental and/or medical specialist.

Align Treatment Plans to Meet Client Needs

In my clinical experience, clients seeking mental health services for anxiety and depression often report recent onset or worsening of bruxing and clenching behaviors. Inquiry typically reveals the presence of tension and/or pain in muscles of the head, neck, back, and jaw/mouth. Some of these clients may have a co-morbid or past diagnosis of TMD, while others may not. Clinical judgment and client preference are vital in developing a treatment plan that meets client needs. Prior to eliciting client preference, it is recommended that the client receive education about the relationship between stress and oral habits, as well as the risks and benefits associated with use of bio-behavioral modalities to address TM-related pain/dysfunction and bruxism. In situations where clients express a desire to address TM-related symptoms as part of their therapeutic sessions, clinicians need to decide which bio-behavioral interventions to use, as well as when and how to integrate them into treatment.

Client Receptiveness to Psychological Treatment

Psychological services for persons with TMDs are most effective when they are open to the view that their symptoms may be related to, or exacerbated by, stress and tension. [8] The difficulties encountered by persons with TMDs during their search for a diagnosis, including the intimation that their symptoms are psychological rather than physical, increase the probability that they will respond to a referral for psychological services with resistance or refusal.

Relapse of Bruxism

Relapse of bruxing behavior is reported to be a problem with TMDs. Studies note that bruxing behaviors may return to their original levels when use of splints or biofeedback is withdrawn. While many authors have portrayed this issue as a general limitation of biofeedback, the short-term effectiveness suggests that the difficulty is not inherent to the modality, but may be related to how treatment gains are (or are not) generalized to daily life (e.g., an external locus of control). Since biofeedback involves use of technology, clients may be more inclined to develop beliefs and attributions about the role of external factors in its beneficial effect, rather than to attribute the benefit to their psychological labor and improved self-efficacy. Additional research in this area is needed. [3,9,47]

Habituation (Biofeedback Therapies)

During biofeedback therapy, studies have reported that patients may habituate to the EMG auditory alarm and fail to awaken when bruxing behaviors are detected during the night. Habituation can be detected by treating clinicians by examining the EMG recordings for long periods of uninterrupted muscular activity. Alarm tones can be adjusted to louder volumes in order to ensure awakenings. [55]

EVALUATION OF CLINICAL OUTCOMES

In clinical settings, psychologists and other mental health professionals often seek to evaluate therapeutic effectiveness. Measures of pain, distress, oral para-functional activities, and masticatory muscle activity are typical targets of these efforts. Relevant psychological factors can also be monitored using commercially available self-report instruments. This section describes the methods used to monitor therapeutic change in persons with TMDs. The type of evaluation chosen by a clinician will depend, in part, on the treatment modality employed (e.g., hypnosis vs. cognitive-behavioral therapy).

Pain Evaluation

Pain intensity has been evaluated using a visual analogue scale (VAS) or categorical scale. With the VAS, pain levels are indicated by the client's mark on a 100 mm line anchored on the left-hand side with "no pain" (0) and on the right-hand side with "worst pain possible" (100). The pain VAS is the distance from the left hand side to the mark indicated (in millimeters). In clinical settings, pain VAS ratings can be recorded during each visit, and in diaries at various time points in the treatment period (e.g., baseline, mid-point, end). Diaries enable patients to provide multiple ratings at different times of day (e.g., morning, afternoon and evening), and have been reported to facilitate client engagement, compliance and treatment acceptability. Facial pain has also been evaluated using a 6-point categorical scale (0=no pain, 5=intense pain) [5,37,42]

Facial discomfort has been assessed using Subjective Units of Distress (SUDS) ratings on an 11-point scale (0, no discomfort; 10, highest discomfort possible). Similar to pain ratings, SUDS can be recorded during each visit and at various points in the treatment. [47]

Both pain ratings and SUDS ratings have demonstrated sensitivity in detecting therapeutic improvement in patients with TMDs.

Qualitative measures, such as pain drawings, make use of a visual schematic so that patients can illustrate the location and qualities of the pain they experience. Multiple views of the face (such as the left, front and right sides) may be particularly helpful. [16]

Electromyography

Electromyography is used either as a primary aspect of behavioral therapy or as a device to evaluate therapeutic change in other therapies. [10,47]

Purchase of, or access to, commercial equipment is required and time is needed for clinicians to acquire the technical knowledge, as well as to train each client to record data. Procedures for configuring the EMG biofeedback device to detect bruxing have been specified and tested. Monitoring periods are required to establish an initial baseline EMG measure prior to treatment, and timeframes of 3 days to 1 week have been used in controlled case studies. [3]

In behavioral therapy protocols, overnight use of the EMG device is required (e.g., 6 to 8 hours). EMG recordings are collected while clients sleep and reflect muscular activity associated with nocturnal clenching and grinding events. The device is configured to produce an auditory alarm that awakens the client when masseter muscle tension exceeds a pre-specified threshold. A threshold of 20 microvolts has been recommended for arousal. Use of the automatic alarm shut-off is not recommended because it interrupts clients' ability to achieve full arousal from sleep. Although EMG devices are calibrated, recordings of the masseter muscle can be distorted by movements of the body, such as yawning, that take place during sleep. [10]

Some studies have made use of EMG recordings from the masticatory muscles (masseter, temporalis) as a way to evaluate therapeutic efficacy. EMG recordings are performed at baseline, during treatment and at the end of a treatment protocol. Clients are required to be attached to the EMG device for a brief period (e.g., 10 minutes) at each evaluation, and typically are placed in a resting position (e.g., sitting in chair). [47]

Psychological Measures

Given the role of cognitive and affective factors that influence pain perception, as well as the role of dispositional personality and coping styles, commercial psychological tests are also useful when evaluating therapeutic progress in persons with TMD. For example, measures of depression, anxiety, anger, and personality have been employed in various studies. In particular, significant therapeutic change in persons with TMDs has been observed with the Brief Symptom Inventory-18. [5,25]

Measures of Mouth Opening & TM Joint Sounds

Measurement of the frequency of sounds in the TM joint and the extent of mouth opening have good fidelity to the clinical criteria required for TMD diagnosis.

Sound frequency has been measured using VAS at each

session (0, none, 100, extreme), as well as a categorical scale at the end of treatment to assess change over time (worse, 1; same, 2; improved, 3; alleviated, 4). [24]

The extent of mouth opening can be measured using self-report (i.e., VAS; 0, none, 100, largest opening imaginable), as well as objective measurement with calipers. Calipers are a useful and relatively non-intrusive device to measure the maximum amount of mouth opening at each treatment session. Successful treatment is associated with increases in maximal mouth opening, and reductions in the frequency of TM joint sounds. The use of calipers may have utility in community health settings but its ease of use, cost and level of acceptability in psychological clinics has not been documented. [23]

In research settings, limitations in jaw use have been measured using The Mandibular Function Impairment Questionnaire. While this instrument has not been commercialized and normative data is not available, it may be of use in clinical settings as a therapeutic monitoring tool. [58]

Para-Functional Habits

Empirical studies have reported use of self-report measures to evaluate the frequency of oral para-functional habits (e.g., nail biting, pen chewing) or bruxing behaviors. These behaviors are often performed without self-awareness, and therefore use of these measures are not reliable estimates of therapeutic change. [5,17] Informant reports (e.g., from family members) may be useful for establishing the presence of para-functional habits or bruxing behaviors in their partner. However, to date, the reliability and validity of informant questionnaires has not been reported in scientific journals.

PRINCIPLES OF EFFECTIVE TREATMENT

Assessment & Mental Health Screening

The chronicity of TMDs places clients at risk for the development of mental health disorders, such as depression and substance abuse. Screening for psychological co-morbidities during intake is valuable.

Cultivate Resilience

Individuals with TMDs consult numerous health care providers in their search for a diagnosis and report that practitioners have a poor understanding of the syndrome. Moreover, they may have chosen unproven treatments that failed to produce any change, or an irreversible procedure that caused lasting physical harm. As such, clients may benefit from therapeutic interventions that cultivate resilience and address feelings of hopelessness. [2,20]

Affordable Community-Based Services

TMD is associated with considerable treatment-related costs. The chronic and relapsing nature of the syndrome necessitates regular use of dental and physical therapies (e.g., massage, physiotherapy, chiropractic), which exhausts third-party insurance coverage, presuming such coverage is available. Moreover, absenteeism and/or reduced availability for work due to TMD symptoms also contribute to financial hardship. Group psychological treatment in community settings may assist with affordability. Knowledge of low-cost or sliding scale treatment programs is helpful.

Use of Bio-behavioral Treatment Modalities

Current best practices in the psychological treatment of TMDs suggest the use of techniques to alleviate pain, reduce stress, promote healthy coping and facilitate relaxation. The most current literature confirms that a number of bio-behavioral modalities are safe and effective in TMDs. [20, 53]

Educate and Mobilize Family and Peer Support

Family and friends play a vital role in motivating persons with TMD to learn new coping skills. Educational resources for TMD syndrome are available (see Resources) and clients may need encouragement to educate loved ones and co-workers about their condition. In-person or online peer support groups may also provide valuable opportunities for clients to meet other individuals with TMDs.

Establish Inter-professional Consultation Procedures

Persons with TMDs typically seek the services of multiple health providers, including physicians, dentists, psychologists, and physical therapists. With the exception of multi-disciplinary pain management clinics that provide services to TMD clients, most clients have to piece together an understanding of the health opinions and treatments of each provider. Inter-professional consultation may be beneficial to evaluate client progress and motivation towards therapeutic goals.

Build Collaborative Professional Partnerships to Address Mental Health Needs

Psychological evaluation is considered to be an important part in the treatment plan for TMDs. Dentists are trained to recognize that psychological factors influence the course and treatment of the problem. Psychologists and other mental health clinicians should consider developing program offerings that embed services directly within or adjacent to dental offices. [7]

Advocacy

A significant proportion of adults and their families are affected by TMD dysfunction. Treatment techniques remain unable to eliminate bruxism and/or pain, and its relapsing course has a negative impact on quality of life. Insurance coverage (even partial) may empower individuals to seek care, and advocacy efforts may be necessary to assist clients in their attempts to obtain funding.

WHAT DO DENTAL GUIDELINES SAY ABOUT PSYCHOSOCIAL TREATMENT?

Dental guidelines for the clinical management of TMDs are vital sources of information for mental health care professionals. They summarize the current perspectives of dental practitioners regarding how psychological interventions can contribute to the overall care of persons with TMD. In this section, the guidelines of four dental associations are reviewed with respect to their recommendations regarding psychosocial care in TMD. The four guidelines are:

1. The American Association of Dental Research Policy Statement on Temporomandibular Disorders (2010)

2. The Royal College of Dental Surgeons of Ontario: Guideline of Diagnosis and Management of Temporomandibular Disorders & Related Musculoskeletal Disorders (2009)

3. American Society of Temporomandibular Joint Surgeons' Guidelines for Diagnosis and Management of Disorders involving the Temporomandibular Joint and Related Musculoskeletal Structures (2003)

4. European Academy of Craniomandibular Disorders: Guidelines and Recommendations for Examination, Diagnosis, Management of Patients with Temporomandibular Disorders and Orofacial Pain by the General Dental Practitioner (2007)

Readers who wish to view these documents in their entirety, or who wish to know more about the procedures used in their development, may consult Appendix A. In many cases, the guidelines are available on the Internet, and links are given in the References section.

1. The American Association of Dental Research Policy Statement on Temporomandibular Disorders (2010)

The American Association for Dental Research (AADR; www.aadronline.org) is a non-profit organization dedicated to the advancement and dissemination of research and knowledge for the purpose of improving oral health. It is a division of the International Association of Dental Research (IADR; www.iadr.org). Membership is composed of dental, oral and craniofacial researchers, including health professionals.

In March 2010, the AADR issued a policy statement regarding the diagnosis and treatment of temporomandibular disorders. [59,60] The policy acknowledged the value of psychosocial assessment of patients with TMDs, including the use of standardized and validated psychometric tests. It also advocated for the use of conservative, reversible and evidence-based treatments, due to their low risk of harm to patients. "Reversible" therapies refer to interventions that reduce symptoms and do not permanently alter the mandibular position or "bite", and include one or more of the following:

- patient education
- relaxation training
- behavioral coping strategies
- patient awareness of clenching and bruxing habits
- physical therapies (e.g., jaw exercises, ultrasound, massage)
- prescription medication (e.g., anti-inflammatories)
- oral appliances (e.g., splints)
- behavioral therapy

Two other dental organizations, the American Academy of Orofacial Pain (www.aaop.org) and the European Academy of Craniomandibular Disorders (www.eacmd.org), endorsed the AADR policy. [61]

2. The Royal College of Dental Surgeons of Ontario: Guideline of Diagnosis and Management of Temporomandibular Disorders & Related Musculoskeletal Disorders (2009)

The Royal College of Dental Surgeons of Ontario (RCDSO) is the governing body for dentists in Ontario (www.rcdso.org). The practice of dentistry in Ontario is regulated by the Dentistry Act (1991) and the Regulated Health Professions Act (1991). Membership in the RCDSO requires the satisfactory completion of educational requirements and licensing exams.

The RCDSO first issued a guideline about the diagnosis and management of TMDs in 1999, which was revised in 2009. [55] The most current guideline [63] outlines the educational requirements of practitioners who assess and treat TMDs, and the clinical responsibilities of providers (e.g., a comprehensive patient history, clinical exam, use of special investigations). With respect to TMD management, the RCDSO acknowledged that "…most TMDs are actually managed rather than definitively treated" and thus, conservative methods are afforded highest priority. The aim of intervention is symptom relief.

RCDSO guidelines indicate that psychological and/or psychiatric treatment (including behavioral modification therapy) is one aspect of a wide range of conservative treatments for TMDs and should be delivered by appropriately qualified practitioners. Other types of conservative treatment include: patient reassurance and education, medications (e.g., anti-inflammatories/analgesics), physical therapy, and trigger point injections (when indicated).

3. American Society of Temporomandibular Joint Surgeons' Guidelines for Diagnosis and Management of Disorders involving the Temporomandibular Joint and Related Musculoskeletal Structures (2003)

The American Society of Temporomandibular Joint Surgeons (ASTJS) is a non-profit organization of maxillofacial, orthopedic, plastic reconstructive and oral surgical specialists dedicated to promoting education, research and patient services concerning orthopedic disease of the temporomandibular joint (www.astmjs.org). Members possess surgical experience and an interest in performing basic or clinical research (e.g., dental specialists, dental surgeons, researchers).

In 2003, the ASTJS issued a guideline about the classification, diagnosis and treatment of TMDs and related disorders. [64] Use of behavior modification is recommended as one of several non-surgical treatment modalities and is to be considered for all symptomatic patients. In particular, the ASTJS recommended that behavioral therapy be focused on helping patients with stress management, including stress-related habits such as bruxism, clenching and gum chewing.

4. European Academy of Craniomandibular Disorders: Guidelines and Recommendations for Examination, Diagnosis, Management of Patients with Temporomandibular Disorders and Orofacial Pain by the General Dental Practitioner (2007)

The European Academy of Craniomandibular Disorders (EACD) is a non-profit organization dedicated to the development of science and education regarding craniomandibular disorders and orofacial pain (www.eacmd.org).

In 2007, the EACD issued a guideline for general dental practitioners with respect to screening for TMD disorders, procedures for assessment and clinical documentation, as well as adult diagnosis and treatment. Additional considerations were provided for children and adolescents. [65]

With respect to psychosocial care, EACD guidelines recommend that general dentists screen for psychosocial factors in patients with TMD and orofacial pain, and inform their patients of the role that these factors may play in their recovery. Referrals to a clinical psychologist or psychotherapist were recommended to clarify these factors and intervene using behavioral, cognitive-behavioral and/or psychological therapy. In particular, EACD recommendations highlight the importance of differentiating patients who have acute vs. chronic pain. Acute pain can be managed using medications and physiotherapy, as well as psychosocial treatments aimed to lower the tension experienced by clients (e.g., stress management). In clients with chronic pain, a referral to a multidisciplinary clinic with experience using strategies to address coping styles, locus of control, and pain management may be indicated. [65]

A WORD ABOUT GUIDELINES FOR CHILDREN AND ADOLESCENTS

Both the EACD and the American Academy of Pediatric Dentistry (AAPD; www.aapd.org) have released guidelines regarding the diagnosis and management of TMDs in children and adolescents. Interested readers may consult the References section for information and links to these documents. [65,66]

SUMMARY

Professional dental guidelines support the use of psychosocial care in the management of TMD. They reflect the science-based understanding that mental disorders (e.g., mood/anxiety disorders) and styles of emotional/behavioral coping influence the functional status and level of pain experienced by persons with TMD. Standardized psychological tests are also valuable in identifying these factors, so that qualified professionals can assist healthcare consumers in ways that enhance their function and build their sense of self-efficacy.

RESOURCES

National Institute of Dental and Craniofacial Research (NIDCR)
www.nidcr.nih.gov/OralHealth/Topics/TMJ/TMJDisorders.htm

According to its mission statement, the NIDCR seeks to improve oral, dental and craniofacial health through research, research training and the dissemination of health information to the public, clinicians, researchers, and policy-makers. This website contains easy-to-read information about the signs/symptoms, diagnosis and treatment of TMDs that are useful for both health specialists and health consumers.

The Canadian Dental Association
www.cda-adc.ca/en/oral_health/talk/complications/temporomandibular_disorder/

Dentists are important care partners in the treatment of bruxism and TMDs. Information on this site is useful for both health specialists and persons with TMDs.

Clinical Trials
www.clinicaltrials.gov
Individuals living in the United States can consult this website for information about clinical trials regarding TMDs.

The Canadian Pain Society
www.canadianpainsociety.ca

The Canadian Pain Society (CPS) is a society of scientists and health professionals with interest in pain research and management. View "Resources" for links to websites with information about pain, pain management and use of opioids. The CPS is a chapter of the International Association for the Study of Pain (IASP), which is a professional forum for science, practice and education in the field of pain. (https://www.iasp-pain.org).

The American Chronic Pain Association (ACPA)
https://theacpa.org

The ACPA has offered peer support and education in pain management skills to people with pain, family and friends, and health care professionals since 1980. Videos and tools to assist doctor-patient conversation about health issues are available directly on the site.

The TMJ Association, Ltd.
www.tmj.org

President and Co-Founder: Terrie Cowley
Founded in 1986, this Wisconsin-based Association offers information to persons with TMDs and their families, and assistance in connecting people via support groups. An e-newsletter is available after registering with the site.

Online Social Support
The Internet has many peer-led support groups on social media sites, such as Twitter and Facebook, which may be of interest to persons with TMDs and their loved ones. Chats and discussion groups can also be found using internet search engines (e.g., Google).

APPENDIX A: HOW ARE PROFESSIONAL GUIDELINES DEVELOPED?

As an author, it has been a pleasure to receive feedback and questions from readers about this book. Increasingly, I am being contacted by readers who have TMDs or TMD-like symptoms, and who do not have any formal training in health or healthcare. They have commented that the medical and psychological terminology is dense. As noted earlier, the aim of this guide is to increase the accessibility of health knowledge about TMDs for practicing clinicians, and so it has been written in a style suited for that audience.

However, in my work as an author and as a Psychologist, I am acutely aware of the challenges to find information about TMDs and options for treatment. While the Internet continues to offer a steady stream of information, the quality and credibility of web content can be difficult to determine. In this book, readers were introduced to two sources of information about the clinical management of TMDs: *clinical practice guidelines* and *policy statements*. Not all readers will be familiar with these types of documents. In this section, readers can learn more about how these documents are prepared, their value for health care practitioners and consumers, and where they can be found on the Internet.

CLINICAL PRACTICE GUIDELINES

A *clinical practice guideline* (CPG) is a written summary of scientific and professional information prepared by a national or international professional organization. It contains information about practices in diagnosis, treatment, educational needs, product development(s), and clients' preferences about care. CPGs are typically read by physicians, specialists, policy makers, hospital administrators, advocacy groups and health care consumers.

Within the health system, CPGs are not viewed as "rules" that health care professionals must follow. Rather, they are used to promote the highest quality of clinical work, to assist consumers in making health-related decisions, and to identify areas in need of future study. [67]

How are CPGs developed?

CPG development starts when a professional organization poses a question about a clinical or health care problem. A multidisciplinary committee of health care providers and researchers who have expertise in health care and scientific methodology is assembled to investigate the evidence related to this problem. [67] The committee conducts a systematic survey of scientific studies published in the past decade (or longer, if needed). [68,69] The process of evidence collection and analysis generates a large "base" upon which recommendations are made. The entire process requires considerable resources of professional time and effort, and may take several years to complete.

Following the survey, a written document is prepared, which includes a summary of health information and recommendations for decision-makers in health settings. The recommendations are accompanied by a "strength rating" that reflects the quality, consistency and amount of supporting evidence, the type of support for each recommendation (e.g., scientific studies, expert opinion, consensus), and the potential for harm to patients (e.g., [70]). The value of a "strength rating" is that readers are explicitly informed about which scientific studies were used to inform a recommendation.

In the last phase of development, intended users of the guidelines (e.g., healthcare consumers, care providers, and administrators of healthcare facilities) are asked to review and provide comment. CPGs may also be subjected to field testing before being finalized. These "external" reviews are valuable because they consider how the recommendations will be implemented and any barriers to doing so. [67] The guideline development committee compiles the "user feedback" and makes a decision about whether recommendations need to be modified.

Following review, the professional organization finalizes and disseminates the CPG by publishing on the Internet, in scientific/professional journals, and by making presentations to hospitals, agencies and government organizations.

How do CPGs help health care consumers?

CPGs offer reliable and accurate health information for consumers who want to learn about their condition, treatment options, and associated risks and benefits of treatment. CPGs also provide an explicit rationale for why certain treatments are preferred, and the factors that influence these choices. Consumers can use the information to prepare for visits with their health care providers, especially when choices are being made about treatment.

One of the disadvantages of CPGs is that readers may not be familiar with the medical terminology contained in them. Some documents may include a plain-language summary to ensure that the information is more accessible to persons without experience or training in the health field.

How do CPGs help healthcare professionals?

Health care professionals use CPGs to stay informed about current developments in health topics. Since CPGs synthesize current scientific findings, they may reduce the risk of ineffective or harmful treatments. If there are controversies about treatments, CPGs make these explicit and facilitate deliberations between professionals.

Are there any negative aspects or disadvantages associated with CPGs?

Concerns have been expressed about the level of quality of CPGs. [67] Although standards have been developed to evaluate the process of guideline development and the quality of reporting (i.e., the AGREE instrument), most health care consumers do not have the tools or skills to evaluate CPG quality. A second disadvantage associated with CPGs is that its recommendations may not be readily taken up in health settings. [68] Thus, consumers who review CPGs may discover that not all the treatment options in the document are actually available.

Given these disadvantages, CPGs are best considered a tool for consumers to educate themselves about their condition and to initiate discussions with care providers. Consumers might consider bringing a copy of CPGs to their visit with a health provider.

How can CPGs be found on the Internet?

There are at least two ways to search for a clinical practice guideline on the Internet:
1. Search websites that have been specifically designed to access CPGs (Table 3) Locate the search window on the site, and type the health condition you are interested in (e.g., temporomandibular disorder).

Table 3: List of Organizations on the Internet with Clinical Practice Guidelines and Search Capability

Organization	Location	Website*
National Guidelines Clearinghouse	USA	http://www.guideline.gov
Canadian Medical Association	Canada	https://www.cma.ca/En/Pages/clinical-practice-guidelines.aspx
UK National Institute for Health and Clinical Evidence	United Kingdom	http://www.nice.org.uk/guidance
Guidelines International Network (GIN)**	Global (based in Scotland)	http://www.g-i-n.net/

* Links verified December 29, 2017.
** Users will need to select "guidelines" to focus their search on the GIN website.

2. Use a general search engine: Enter the phrase "clinical practice guideline" and the name of the health condition (e.g., temporomandibular disorder, fibromyalgia, etc.) in a web-based search engine (e.g., www.google.ca).

POLICY STATEMENTS

Policy statements are another source of information about health conditions that are written by professional organizations and available to the public. Policies are written to express an official position of an organization on an issue, and to inform members and their stakeholders about future activities of the organization (e.g., legislation, advocacy, regulation).

How are policy statements developed?

Like CPGs, policy statements are prepared by professional organizations that assemble a committee of health care practitioners and researchers to answer a question about a health problem. Scientific studies are reviewed and a written statement is prepared. Draft policy statements are usually approved by an executive council of the professional organization before they are released. References to the scientific studies are included in the policy.

Policy statements are documents that reflect the values and opinions of the organization that prepared them, so they do not include "strength ratings" for their recommendations and "user feedback" is not requested from external stakeholders. While policy statements intend to reflect the views of an entire organization, participation in a professional organization is voluntary, and individual members may disagree with written organizational policies.

How do policy statements help health care consumers?

Policy statements are produced by organizations for the purpose of informing other organizations about their position on a health issue. These documents are helpful for consumers to understand what activities these organizations support, and their position on legislation or regulation. These statements can be particularly helpful when the management of a condition is controversial, when there are a wide range of treatment options, or when there is evidence that past treatments have caused harm to consumers. After reading a policy statement, consumers may wish to ask their health care providers about whether they are a member of that organization and whether they agree or disagree with the policy.

How do policy statements help healthcare professionals?

Policy statements are reflective of a professional organization's point of view regarding the kinds of change they see as necessary to improve future health care for a condition. Health care professionals (who may or may not be members of the organization) may agree or disagree with the views expressed, and their perspectives may be written in a published scientific journal or in the reports of association meetings. When policy statements are controversial, meetings may be arranged at scientific conferences or association meetings so that members can discuss their views.

Are there any negative aspects or disadvantages associated with policy statements?

In professional settings, there is no explicit expectation that the opinions in policy statements will be implemented in a doctor's office. As a result, the information contained in them may be more aspirational in intent, and may not reflect the practices that are currently being used in the offices of health care providers.

How can policy statements be found on the Internet?

To locate a policy statement on the Internet, enter the phrase "policy statement" and the name of the health condition (e.g., temporomandibular disorder, fibromyalgia, etc.) in a search engine (e.g., www.google.com). These search terms may also be entered into databases such as Pubmed (http://www.ncbi.nlm.nih.gov/pubmed). For assistance using search engines, contact a librarian at your local library or at a nearby college or university.

REFERENCES

1. Brooke, R.I., Stenn, P.G., & Mothersill, K.J. (1977). The diagnosis and conservative treatment of myofascial pain dysfunction syndrome. *Oral Surgery, Oral Medicine, and Oral Pathology, 44*(6), 844-52.

2. Garro, L.C., Stephenson, K.A., & Good, B.J. (1994). Chronic illness of the temporomandibular joints as experienced by support-group members. *Journal of General Internal Medicine, 9,* 372-378.

3. Moss, R.A., Garrett, J. & Chiodo, J.F. (1982). Temporo-mandibular joint dysfunction and myofascial pain dysfunction syndrome: Parameters, etiology and treatment. *Psychological Bulletin, 92,* 331-346.

4. Simon, E.P., & Lewis, D.M. (2000). Medical hypnosis for temporomandibular disorders: Treatment efficacy and medical utilization outcome. *Oral Surgery, Oral Medicine, Oral Pathology, Oral Radiology, and Endodontics, 90,* 54-63.

5. Glaros, A.G., & Glass, E.G. (1993). Temporomandibular disorders. In R.J. Gatchel, & E.B. Blanchard (Eds.), *Psychophysiological Disorders: Research and Clinical Applications* (p.299-356). Washington, D.C.: American Psychological Association.

6. Hansson, T., & Nilner, M. (1975). A study of the occurrence of symptoms of diseases of the TMJ, masticatory musculature, and related structures. *Journal of Oral Rehabilitation, 2,* 239-243.

7. Jerolimov, V. (2009). Temporomandibular disorders and orofacial pain. *Medical Sciences, 33,* 53-77.

8. Garro, L.C. (1994). Narrative representations of chronic illness experience: Cultural models of illness, mind, and body in stories concerning the temporomandibular joint (TMJ). *Social Science and Medicine, 38*(6), 775-788.

9. Morse, D.R. (2014). Stress and Bruxism: A Critical Review and Report of Cases. *Journal of Human Stress, 8*(1), 43-54.

10. Cherasia, M., & Parks, L. (1986). Suggestions for use of behavioral measures in treating bruxism. *Psychological Reports, 58*, 719-722.

11. Watson, T.S. (1993). Effectiveness of arousal and arousal plus overcorrection to reduce nocturnal bruxism. *Journal of Behavioral Therapy and Experimental Psychiatry, 24*, 181-185.

12. Moss, R.A., Ruff, M.H. & Sturgis, E.T. (1984). Oral behavioral patterns in facial pain, headache and non-headache populations. *Behavior Research and Therapy, 22*(6), 683-687.

13. Tsai, C.-M., Chou, S.-L., Gale, E.N., McCall, W.D. (2002). Human masticatory muscle activity and jaw position under experimental stress. *Journal of Oral Rehabilitation, 32*, 584-588.

14. Glaros, A.G. & Rao, S.M. (1979). Electromyographic correlates of experimentally-induced stress in diurnal bruxists and normals. *Journal of Dental Research, 58*(9), 1872-1878.

15. Glaros, A.G. & Rao, S.M. (1977). Bruxism: A Critical Review. *Psychological Bulletin, 84*(4), 76-781.

16. Peterson, A.L., Dixon, D.C., Talcott, G.W., & Kelleher, W.J. (1993). Habit reversal treatment of temporomandibular joint disorders: A pilot investigation. *Journal of Behavioral Therapy and Experimental Psychiatry, 24*, 49-55.

17. Wojnilover, D.A. & Gross, L.M. (1981). The treatment of bruxism: A review and proposal for research. *Clinical Psychology Review, 1,* 453-468.

18. Nadler, S.C. (1957). Bruxism, a classification: Critical review. *Journal of the American Dental Association, 54,* 615-622.

19. Laskin, D.M. (1969). Etiology of the pain-dysfunction syndrome. *American Dental Association, 79,* 147-153.

20. Laskin, D.M. & Block, S. (1986). Diagnosis and treatment of myofascial pain-dysfunction (MPD) syndrome. *The Journal of Prosthetic Dentistry, 56*(1), 75-84.

21. Carvalho, A.L., Cury, A.A., Garcia, R.C. (2008). Prevalence of bruxism and emotional stress and the association between them in Brazilian police officers. *Brazilian Oral Research, 22*(1), 31-5.

22. Manfredini, D., Landi, N., Fantoni, F., Segu, M. & Bosco, M. (2005). Anxiety symptoms in clinical diagnosed bruxers. *Journal of Oral Rehabilitation, 32,* 584-588.

23. Manfredini, D., Ciapparelli, A. Dell'Osso, L, & Bosco, M. (2005). Mood disorders in subjects with bruxing behavior. *Journal of Dentistry, 33,* 485-490.

24. Stam, H.J., McGrath, P.A., & Brooke, R.I. (1984). The effects of a cognitive-behavioral treatment program on temporo-mandibular pain and dysfunction syndrome. *Psychosomatic Medicine, 46*(6), 534-545.

25. Ferrando, M., Galdon, M.J., Dura, E., Andreau, Y., Jimenez, Y., & Poveda, R. (2012). Enhancing the efficacy of treatment for temporomandibular patients with muscular diagnosis through cognitive-behavioral intervention, including hypnosis: a randomized study. *Oral Surgery, Oral Medicine, Oral Pathology, and Oral Radiology, 113,* 81-89.

26. Gatchel, R.J., Garofalo, J.P., Ellis, E. & Holt, C. (1996). Major psychological disorders in acute and chronic TMD: An initial examination. *Journal of the American Dental Association, 127*, 1365-1374.

27. Kight, M., Gatchel, R.J., & Wesley, L. (1999). Temporomandibular Disorders: Evidence for Significant Overlap with Psychopathology. *Health Psychology, 18*(2), 177-182.

28. Kinney, R.K., Gatchel, R.J., Ellis, E. & Holt, C. (1992). Major psychological disorders in chronic TMD patients: Implications for successful management. *Journal of the American Dental Association, 123*, 49-54.

29. Korszun, A., Hinderstein, B., & Wong, M. (1996). Comorbidity of depression with chronic facial pain and temporomandibular disorders. *Oral Surgery, Oral Medicine, Oral Pathology, Oral Radiology and Endodontology, 82*(5), 496-500.

30. McCracken, L.M. & Gatchel, R.J. (2000). The magnification of psychopathology sequelae associated with multiple chronic medical conditions. *Journal of Applied Biobehavioral Research, 5*(1), 92-99.

31. Riley, J.L. & King, C. (2009). Self-report of alcohol use for pain in a multi-ethnic community sample. *Journal of Pain, 10*, 944-952. doi: 10.1016/j.jpain.2009.03.005.

32. Nicholas, M. K., & Wright, M. (2001). Management of acute and chronic pain. In J. Milgrom & G.D. Burrows (Eds.) *Psychology and psychiatry: Integrating medical practice.* (pp. 127-153). New York: John Wiley & Sons Ltd.

33. Fischer, W.F. & O'toole, E.T. (1993). Personality characteristics of chronic bruxers. *Behavioral Medicine, 19*, 82-86.

34. Schneider, C., Schaefer, R., Ommerborn, M.A., Giraki, M., Boertz, A., Raab, W., & Franz, M., (2007). Maladaptive coping strategies in patients with bruxism compared to non-bruxing controls. *International Journal of Behavioral Medicine, 14,* 257-261.

35. Woods, D.W., & Miltenberger, R.G. (1995). Habit reversal: A review of applications and variations. *Journal of Behavior Therapy and Experimental Psychiatry, 26*(2), 123-131.

36. Azrin, N.H., & Nunn, R.G. (1973). Habit reversal: A method of eliminating nervous habits and tics. *Behaviour Research and Therapy, 11,* 619- 628.

37. Rosenbaum, M.S. & Ayllon, T. (1981). Treating bruxism with the habit reversal technique. *Behavior Research & Therapy, 19,* 87-96

38. Gramling, S.E., Neblett, J., Grayson, R., & Townsend, D. (1996). Temporomandibular disorder: Efficacy of an oral habit reversal treatment program. *Journal of Behavioral Therapy and Experimental Psychology, 27*(3), 245-255.

39. Azrin, N.H., & Peterson, A.L. (1990). Treatment of Tourette Syndrome by habit reversal: A waiting-list control group comparison. *Behaviour Therapy, 21,* 305-318.

40. Glaros, A.G., Kim-Weroha, N., Lausten, L., & Franklin, K.L. (2007). Comparison of habit reversal and a behaviorally-modified dental treatment for temporomandibular disorders: A pilot investigation. *Applied Psychophysiology and Biofeedback, 32,* 149-154.

41. Townsend, D., Nicholson, R.A., Buenaver, L., Bush,, F., & Gramling, S. (2001). Use of a habit reversal treatment for temporomandibular pain in a minimal therapist contact format. *Journal of Behavior Therapy, 32,* 221-239.

42. Teleska, J., & Roffman, A. (2004). A continuum of hypnotherapeutic interactions: From formal hypnosis to hypnotic conversation. *American Journal of Clinical Hypnosis, 47*, 103-115.

43. Elkins, G., Jensen, M.P., & Patterson, D.R. (2007). Hypnotherapy for the management of chronic pain. *International Journal of Clinical and Experimental Hypnosis, 55*, 275-287.

44. Crasilneck, H.B. (1995). The use of the Crasilneck Bombardment Technique in Problems of Intractable Organic Pain. *American Journal of Clinical Hypnosis, 37*, 255-266.

45. Golan, H.P. (1989). Temporomandibular joint disease treated with hypnosis. *American Journal of Clinical Hypnosis, 31*, 269-274.

46. LaCrosse, M.B. (1994). Understanding change: Five-year follow-up of brief hypnotic treatment of chronic bruxism. *American Journal of Clinical Hypnosis, 36*, 276-281.

47. Somer, E. (1991). Hypnotherapy in the treatment of chronic nocturnal use of a dental splint described for bruxism. *The International Journal of Clinical and Experimental Hypnosis, 24*, 145-154.

48. Stolzenberg, J. (1953). Case reports on bruxism and periodic hysterical trismus. *Journal of Clinical and Experimental Hypnosis, 1*, 67 – 70. doi: 10.1080/00207145308410939

49. Winocur, E., Gavish, A., Emodi-Perlman, A., Halachmi, M., & Eli, I. (2002). Hypnorelaxation as treatment for myofascial pain disorder: A comparative study. *Oral Surgery, Oral Medicine, Oral Pathology, Oral Radiology, and Endodontics, 93*, 429-34.

50. Orlando, B. Manfredini, D., Salvetti, G., & Bosco, M. (2007). Evaluation of the effectiveness of biobehavioral therapy in the treatment of temporomandibular disorders: A literature review. *Behavioral Medicine, 33*(3), 101-118.

51. Jacobson E. (1938) Progressive Relaxation (2nd ed). University of Chicago Press, Chicago.

52. Bourne, E.J. (2010). The Anxiety & Phobia Workbook. California: New Harbinger Publications.

53. Dworkin, S.F. (1997). Behavioral and educational modalities. *Oral Surgery, Oral Medicine, Oral Pathology, Oral Radiology, and Endodontics, 83,* 128-33.

54. Rollman, G.B. & Gillespie, J.M. (2000). The role of psychosocial factors in temporomandibular disorders. *Current Review of Pain, 4,* 71-81.

55. Moss, R.A., Hammer, D., Adams, H.E., Jenkins, J.O., Thompson, K., & Haber, J. (1982). A more efficient biofeedback procedure for the treatment of nocturnal bruxism. *Journal of Oral Rehabilitation, 9,* 125-131.

56. Stenn, P.G., Mothersill, K.J., & Brooke, R.I. (1979). Biofeedback and a cognitive behavioral approach to treatment of myofascial pain dysfunction syndrome. *Oral Surgery, Oral Medicine, and Oral Pathology, 44*(6), 844-52.

57. Dworkin, S.F., Turner, J.A., Wilson, L., Massoth, D., Whitney, C., Huggins, K.H., … & Truclove, E. (1994). Brief group cognitive-behavioral intervention for temporomandibular disorders. *Pain, 59,* 175-187.

58. Stegenga, B., de Bont, L.G.M., de Leeuw, R., & Boering, G. (1993). Assessment of mandibular function impairment associated with temporomandibular joint osteoarthrosis and internal derangement. *Journal of Orofacial Pain, 7,* 183–195.

59. Greene, C.S. (2010). Managing the care of patients with temporomandibular disorders: A new guideline for care. *Journal of the American Dental Association, 141*(9), 1086-8.

60. American Association for Dental Research (2015). Policy Statement on Temporomandibular Disorders. Retrieved from http://www.aadronline.org/i4a/pages/index.cfm?pageid=3465#.VdnX4rTHKREA on November 12, 2015. Current Link accessed at http://www.iadr.org/AADR/About-Us/Policy-Statements/Science-Policy#TMD on December 29, 2017.

61. Greene, C.S. (2010) Letters from those who take issue with AADR's revised policy and Dr. Greene's statement: author reply. *Journal of the American Dental Association, 141*(12), 1416-7.

62. Greene, C.S., Klasser, G.D., & Epstein, J.B. (2010). Revision of the American Association of Dental Research's Science Information Statement about Temporomandibular Disorders. *Journal of the Canadian Dental Association, 76*, a115.

63. Royal College of Dental Surgeons of Ontario. (2009). Guidelines: Diagnosis and Management of Temporomandibular Disorders & Related Musculoskeletal Disorders. Toronto: Royal College of Dental Surgeons of Ontario. Accessed at http://www.rcdso.org/KnowledgeCentre/RCDSOLibrary (Professional practice > Guidelines) on September 1, 2015.

64. American Society of Temporomandibular Joint Surgeons. (2003). Guidelines for diagnosis and management of disorders involving the temporomandibular joint and related musculoskeletal structures. *Cranio 21*, 68-76.

65. DeBoever, J.A., Nilner, M., Orthlief, J-D., Steenks, M.H. & Educational Committee of the European Academy of Craniomandibular Disorders. (2007). Recommendations for examination, diagnosis, managements of patients with Temporomandibular disorders and orofacial pain by the general dental practitioner. *Journal of Orofacial Pain 22*(3), 268-278. Accessed on November 16, 2015 at http://www.eacmd.org/gpguidelines.php

66. American Academy of Pediatric Dentistry (2010). Guidelines on acquired temporomandibular disorders in infants, children and adolescents. Chicago (Il): American Academy of Pediatric Dentistry (AAPD). 6 p. Retrieved from http://www.aapd.org/media/Policies_Guidelines/G_TMD .pdf on August 23, 2015.

67. Brouwers, M., Stacey, D., & O'Connor, A. (2013). Knowledge translation tools. In S. Straus, J. Tetroe, D. Graham (Eds). *Knowledge Translation in Health Care: Moving from Evidence to Practice.* (pp. 50-62). Second Edition. New Jersey, USA: John Wiley & Sons, Ltd.

68. Harrison, M.B., Légaré, F., Graham, I.D., & Fevers, B. (2010). Adapting clinical practice guidelines to local context and assessing barriers to their use. *Canadian Medical Association Journal, 182*(2), E78-E84.

69. Kitto, S., Bell, M., Peller, J., Sargeant, J., Etchells, E., Reeves, S., & Silver, I. (2013). Positioning continuing education: boundaries and intersections between the domains continuing education, knowledge translation, patient safety and quality improvement. *Advances in Health Science Education, 18,* 141-156.

70. Fantl, J.A., Newman, D.K., Colling, J., DeLancey, J.O.L., Keeys, C., Loughery, R., … Whitmore, K. (1996). Urinary Incontinence in Adults: Acute and Chronic Management. Clinical Practice Guideline No. 2 (96-0682). Rockville, MD: U.S. Department of Health and Human Services.